Clean Eating:

The Revolutionary Way

to Keeping Your Body

Lean and Healthy

By Amelia Simons

Table of Contents

Introduction

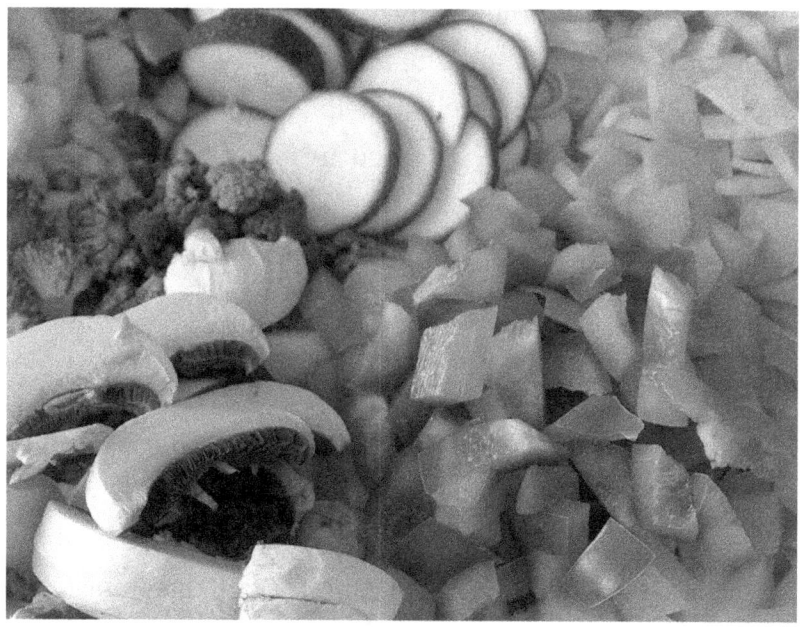

We live in a fast-paced environment. Our society practices and values multi-tasking and always being on the go. If you don't act and move just as fast as the rest of the crowd, you'll probably be considered as an underachiever or, worse yet, just plain lazy. These days, society considers multi-tasking as synonymous with productivity. While this may be true for some, this busyness can often result in people losing their greatest asset– their health.

Fast-paced living has paved the way for people to resort to processed food and fast food meals for convenience. This behavior is good for businesses selling fast foods but not for the consumers themselves. According to several studies in the literature, the availability and the abundance of processed foods have caused people to wreak havoc on their health. These studies suggest that these types of foods are high in trans fat, sodium, and sugar. These substances make food more palatable and help extend the foods' shelf life. However, they are not good for your health, and the increased incidence of heart disease, diabetes, and cancer can attest to that.

So, what can be done to change this?

Learning how to eat healthy can change these studies dramatically. No matter how much you try to work out in a week, you still cannot achieve optimum health if you eat the wrong kinds of food. It is for this reason that more and more people are searching for healthier eating program. One of the results that came from a desire to eat better is the Clean Eating diet.

Clean eating has attracted a number of loyal followers since it was established--many like you who are searching for healthier ways to eat. To help you with your research, this book will explore many of the aspects involved with the Clean Eating Program.

By the end of this book, you will have gained knowledge about what this program is about, its benefits, and how you can begin to eat this way. So, welcome to **Clean Eating** and a healthier lifestyle.

What Is Clean Eating?

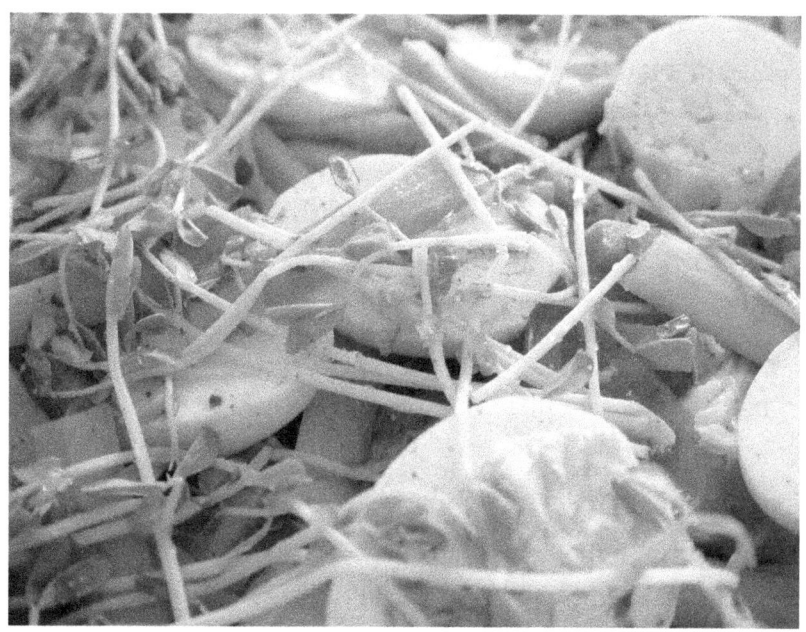

In recent years, there has been a surge of diet plans and programs. This is in response to the increasing consciousness of people desiring to lose weight and improve their overall health. This has resulted in an increase in the number of "healthy" eating plans and programs. Ironically, at the same time, there has been an escalating incidence of heart problems, diabetes, and other lifestyle diseases. However, one of the programs that is making a name for itself in the health and wellness industry is the clean eating program.

What Is Clean Eating?

Clean eating does not directly pertain to the cleanliness of food. Instead, it focuses more directly on how food is prepared. In contrast to other eating plans, this program is not specifically designed for people who want simply to lose weight. In fact, the experts in this area proclaim it is not a diet at all, but instead a lifestyle. This program is about eating food in its most natural form--whole, unrefined and unprocessed food. (Unprocessed foods are those that contain little to no preservatives at all.)

The basic idea of clean eating is not new. In fact, the principle behind this program is rooted in the natural health movement from the 1960s. Clean Eating encompasses the consumption of whole foods like fruits, vegetables, lean meats, healthy fats, and complex carbohydrates, while also promoting the consumption of unprocessed food.

Although the idea behind this eating program has been around for quite some time, it was not widely known until Tosca Reno, a Canadian fitness model, published a series of clean eating cookbooks. While the principles remain the same as they were with the natural health movement in the 1960s, Reno has helped to popularize this eating program.

Clean eating is for people who want to make intelligent and healthy eating choices, who want to become fit, who desire to feel better, and who feel a need to limit their intake of processed foods. Because this eating program is aimed toward the consumption of foods in their most natural state, eating this way will enable your body to function at its best and as a result, can help you feel fantastic and full of energy.

What It Is Not

If you are looking for another fad diet, then clean eating is not for you. Proponents of this program make it clear that this is not a diet but more of a way of life. If you are overweight, it is a program that can help you lose those extra pounds as well as helping those who need to gain weight so their bodies can be healthy.

Unlike other eating programs that you already know about, it does not require you to starve yourself or cause you to have to count things like calories, points, carbs, grams, and fat. You do not have to buy pre-packaged or pre-portioned food, and you are not required to take pills or special potions. What this eating program calls for is consciously deciding to make the choice of choosing and eating whole and natural foods.

The Basics of Clean Eating

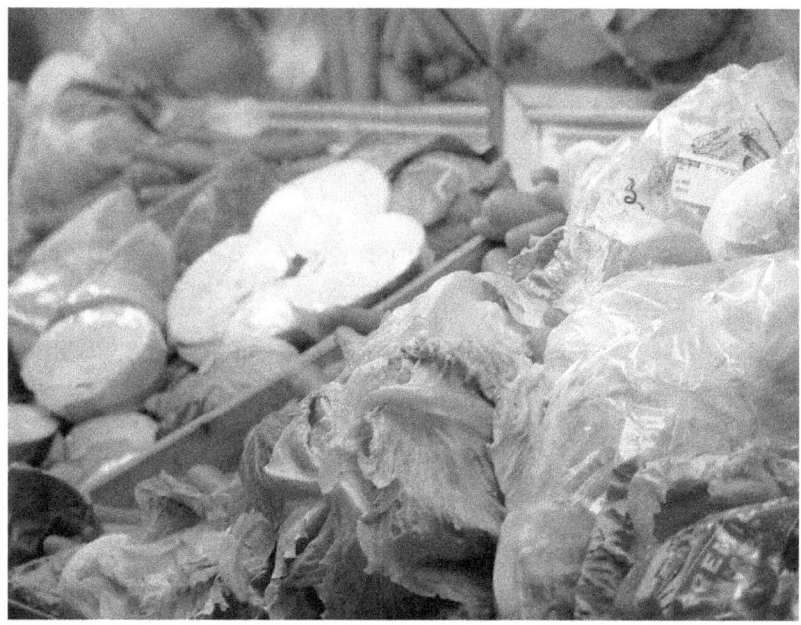

If you have been keeping up with the latest trends in health, then you have probably read some things about clean eating. As I have mentioned earlier, clean eating is not a diet, but instead is a lifestyle choice. Unlike fad diets, clean eating does not promise that you will lose weight, nor does it promote counting calories or points. However, what it does do is encourage healthy eating.

To get started with your very own clean eating program, it is important to get to know the basics:

1. Fruits and Vegetables

Fruits and vegetables are important elements of this eating program. While they are not the central focus, the consumption of these foods is a vital part of healthy eating.

Fruits and vegetables are important for their cleansing and detoxifying properties. For instance, kale has detoxifying properties while celery eliminates excess fluids from the body. Apples also have healing compounds that get rid of carcinogenic toxins in the body while lemons can eliminate putrefactive bacteria and mucous buildup in the intestines.

2. Lean Proteins

Other than fruits and vegetables, this program encourages a diet comprised of lean proteins. This would include plant-based proteins that are low in fat and high in fiber. Examples of plant-based proteins include beans, legumes, tofu, and other soy-based products. Other sources of lean proteins include white meat poultry, fish, and lean cuts of beef.

Lean proteins are excellent sources of B vitamins, such as niacin and riboflavin, iron, magnesium, zinc, and vitamins E and C. B vitamins can help raise your energy levels and improve nervous system function while zinc helps the immune system function normally.

3. Whole Grains

Because clean eating is about eating foods in their most basic form, this includes the presence of whole grains. Whole grains are unprocessed foods that have a higher concentration of fiber and protein than their processed counterpart. Whole grains are good sources of energy but are low in saturated fat. Examples of whole grains are bread, oatmeal, wheat germ, flaxseed, brown rice, and whole-wheat pasta.

Whole grains are extremely popular in many dietary programs because they can help a dieter maintain weight and improve their health. According to various studies, whole grains can help carotid arteries become healthier and reduce the risk of a variety of medical conditions such as colorectal cancer, heart problems, gum disease, and hypertension.

4. Water

Other than healthy and natural food sources, another important part of clean eating is consuming water on a daily basis. Unlike soda and other sugar-laden drinks, water has zero calories and does not contain any sugar. It helps regulate the body's functions and aids in improving one's metabolism. An intake of eight glasses or more of water per day is advised.

Drinking the recommended amount of water per day can help you keep a healthy balance of fluids in your body. It can help you maintain the right body temperature as well as improve circulation and transportation of nutrients throughout your body.

5. Healthy Snacks

Forget about cookies, chips, and cakes. Clean eating is not about consuming these types of snacks because they are high in saturated fat. Instead of pastries that are high in fat and drinks that are overloaded with sugar, the clean eating promotes healthy snacks such as fruits, nuts, vegetables, whole grain crackers, and low-fat milk or yogurt.

If, along the way, you find yourself still confused about what foods to eat or avoid, strive for food choices that are edible in their most natural state like apples, oranges, nuts, seeds, whole grains, and vegetables.

The Benefits of Eating Clean

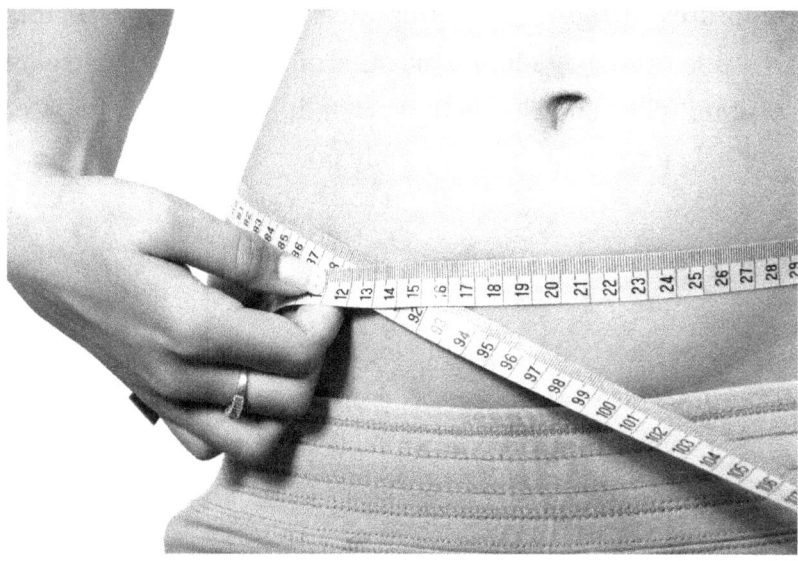

Since the day it was made public, the Clean Eating program became a hit. Its popularity did not just spread among the health-conscious crowd but also among those who are looking for ways to change their eating habits as well. Although the principle behind this program has been practiced since the 1960s, the idea has only come out more recently.

It's no surprise why this eating program has been gaining a lot of positive feedback, and the number of followers continues to grow. The benefits of Clean Eating have surpassed those that have been claimed by different fad diets, even the most famous ones. Here are some of the benefits of eating clean:

Healthy Weight

Advocates of the Clean Eating diet made it clear that this isn't one of those fad diets out there. Those who are trying to slim down can achieve their weight loss goals as the diet is widely known to decrease body fat.

The program is also not just for those who want to shed extra fat but also those who want to gain weight. The diet promotes the consumption of foods in their most natural state, and this enables the body to function how it normally should. When the body functions well, it achieves a healthy weight.

Those who want to maintain a healthy weight can also benefit from this clean eating lifestyle. You will not regain the weight you lost by continually consuming healthy foods recommended in this program.

Improved Energy Level

The most common source of body's energy is glucose. Glucose comes from the food you eat, particularly from carbohydrates. Carbohydrates are divided into two groups: complex and simple.

In contrast to simple carbohydrates, complex carbohydrates make you feel full longer because they are composed of both starch and fiber. It takes some time for the body to process complex carbs. Sources of complex carbohydrates such as whole grains, starchy vegetables, and legumes result to a sustained release of energy.

By getting into the Clean Eating diet, you will be able to improve your energy level. You will no longer be lethargic and will have sufficient energy to keep you going the entire day.

Healthy Skin and Hair

You don't have to spend too much money experimenting on products to fight acne, wrinkles, and look younger. Because Clean Eating promotes sufficient intake of water, it will help you achieve healthier skin. Aside from hydration, water flushes out toxins, giving you that natural glow. Since you don't consume high-glycemic foods such as processed sugar in this diet, you will be less susceptible to acne and breakouts.

The fruits and vegetables that you would be eating in this diet can also help you grow healthy hair. Consuming sufficient amounts of water can also hydrate, eliminate impurities and strengthen your hair.

Stronger Immune System

Your overall health condition will improve once you follow this program. The fruits, vegetables, yogurt and fermented food that you will consume can significantly help maintain a healthy number of probiotics in your digestive system.

Probiotics can regulate your immune system response and make it healthy.

Reduced Risk of Lifestyle Diseases

The risk for having lifestyle diseases such as hypertension, stroke, and diabetes will be greatly reduced with this Clean Eating program. These diseases often stem from unhealthy foods such as those that contain sodium, fat, and sugar-laden food products, and practices such as sedentary lifestyle and smoking. You will consume less artificial food additives, sugar, preservatives, and pesticides, which are the most popular causes of life-threatening conditions such as cancer.

Better Sleep

The vitamins and minerals contained in the whole foods you consume in this diet can help regulate hormonal function. Healthy foods have calming effects on your nervous system and can help trigger a response of sleep-inducing hormone production. All of these can promote better sleep especially during night time. You are less likely to have difficulties sleeping at night and have insomnia.

Saves Money

Unlike fad diets, the Clean Eating program helps you to save more money. Processed and fast foods or those that are pre-packaged are not just unhealthy, but they will also cost you more than their homemade versions. Since you will become healthier, you will be less prone to illnesses that require costly medications. This will save you from spending on treatments and surgical procedures that are needed to help you recover from ailments.

Lifetime Effects

The weight management and health effects offered by this program can last a lifetime. It is not like other dietary programs that are to be followed for a certain period. You can practice clean eating your entire life, and this means that you will also get permanent benefits.

Environment-Friendly

These foods or food groups have the least impact in the environment because less energy is used and lesser waste is produced from them.

These are just among the many benefits of eating clean. These results will vary from one person to another depending on the body's response, but overall, these are the most common benefits provided by the program.

16

Rules of Clean Eating

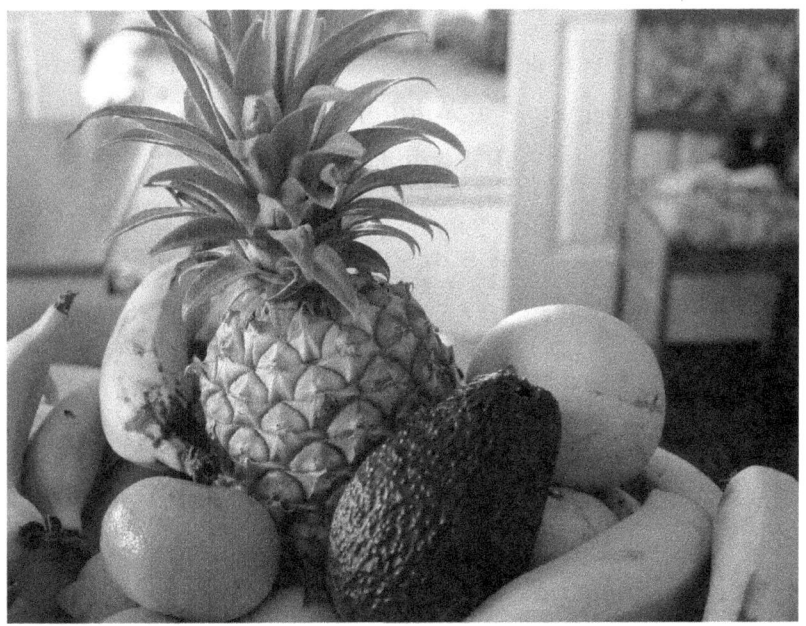

If you haven't tried any form of eating program before, the principle of Clean Eating might seem overwhelming for you. It may sound complex, but looking at its core principle, you will find out that it's very simple. Incorporating the Clean Eating program into your regular lifestyle can be easy. To help you get started with it, here are the rules of Clean Eating:

1. Focus on fresh produce

These include fruits and vegetables grown organically if possible. Aside from needed vitamins and minerals, fruits and vegetables also provide you with dietary fiber, needed for flushing out waste and toxins from your body. This natural product can help you feel healthier and better.

Although you can still get nutrients by consuming health-promoting supplements, doing it will make you feel hungrier and deprived. It will make you cheat and resort to eating unhealthy foods impulsively just to satisfy your hunger. Find the best-tasting fruits and vegetables that are in season and make it a habit to consume them.

2. Avoid processed foods

Processed foods are often loaded with artificial flavoring, sodium, sugar and saturated fats. While some of these substances help in prolonging the food's shelf life and improve their palatability, they won't do anything good for your health. Clean Eating keeps you from consuming this kind of food product. You should also avoid consumption of refined foods such as white bread as they are less healthy options.

The processed foods that you should avoid include canned foods as they have huge amounts of fat and sodium. You should also avoid eating pasta meals that are not made of whole grains. You also should not eat packaged snack foods such as chips, frozen dinners which are high in sodium, sugary breakfast cereals, processed meats, and boxed meal mixes.

3. Eat 5–6 meals in a day

Several studies have already been conducted regarding the benefits of having more than 3 meals a day. According to these studies, having small, frequent meals in a day could help in maintaining a healthy weight and even promote weight loss for those who are overweight. This is because eating more than three times a day could help you curb your cravings. However, this should be done with certain considerations – one of which is to make sure that every meal is healthy. So, it would be a no-no to eat sugar- and salt-laden meals.

4. Have a balanced meal

What sets the Clean Eating program from other eating programs out there is that it focuses more on nutrition than the idea of making you lose weight. One of the key rules of Clean Eating is to eat a balanced meal on a daily basis. It won't restrict you from carbohydrates or fats. Instead, it motivates you to choose healthier alternatives like choosing complex over simple carbs and healthy fats as opposed to trans fats. You can consume unsaturated fats such as omega-3 and omega-6 fatty acids.

5. Drink more water

The importance of a sufficient intake of water has been stressed by health gurus for decades now. Aside from hydrating your body, water helps in maintaining normal body processes. Drinking sufficient amounts of water is also necessary for those who are working out. According to research, water plays a significant role in the growth of muscles and the prevention of catabolism.

6. Check the ingredients

Learn to read food labels. Avoid food products with ingredients that you can't read. If it bears ingredients that you can hardly read, pronounce, or understand, then it's better to ditch that food. Clean Eating is all about food simplicity, and this means that you need to consume foods that have minimal or no additives. It is also best that you avoid purchasing products that contain 5 to 6 ingredients or more. Products with a long list of ingredients are often unhealthy and heavily processed.

7. Approach each meal as part of your lifestyle

One of the best things about the Clean Eating program is that it's sustainable. This means that you can do it for life, regardless of whether or not you want to lose weight. If you want to be part of this revolutionary eating program, then be prepared to change your approach to food. Try to consider clean eating as something that you can practice for the rest of your life.

8. Prioritize the nutrients

Your clean-eating plan should focus more on nutrients than calories. Of course, it is important to measure your caloric intake. However, it is not becoming thin that makes you healthy but having the right body weight. You can achieve and maintain the right weight if you focus on nourishing your body with the right amount of nutrients it needs. Satisfying your nutritional needs can positively affect your weight and health.

You should stop thinking about calories or point counting as there is no need to do so here. All that you are required to do is to settle with natural and healthy produce and consider eating them regularly.

Should You Follow the Eat Clean Diet?

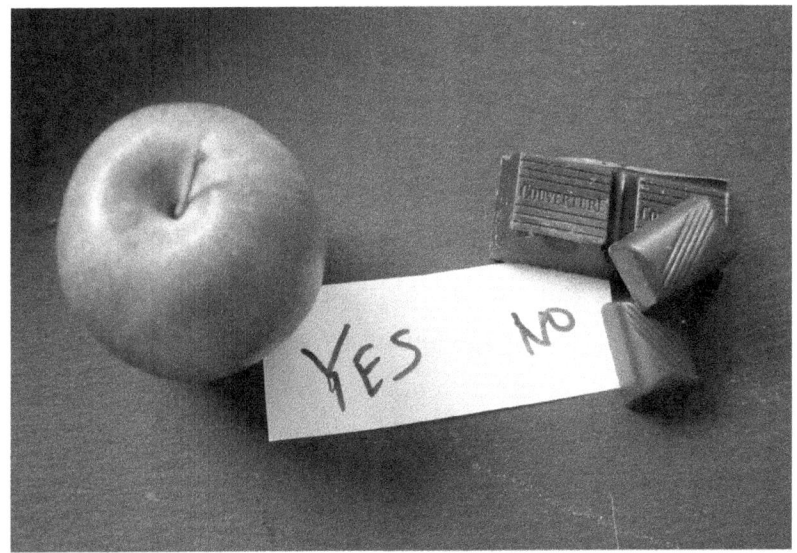

Clean Eating has become synonymous with healthy eating. This is thanks to the series of Clean Eating books released by Tosca Reno, a bestselling author, columnist, motivational speaker, and consultant. With the increasing popularity of this eating program comes the question, "Will it work for everybody?"

This skepticism is totally understandable. Although the advocates of this eating program stress that it isn't a diet, history has shown that not all people respond the same way to diets or eating programs. Some have a positive response, while there are also those who have minimal or no favorable response at all.

How the Eat Clean Diet Works

The Eat Clean diet works through its promotion of natural produce and whole grain products, combined with physical activity and calorie-controlled meals. It involves eating foods in their natural state and taste. When the body takes high quality food, it apparently becomes stronger and healthier. If it is fuelled with low-grade food, it will become weak and more susceptible to illnesses. This diet ensures that your body will only be taking foods that can make your internal organs work at their best. Since these foods are rich in nutrients and do not contain harmful substances, your body will only receive the vitamins and minerals it needs.

This eating program is comprised of the following key points: 80% food, 10% exercise, and 10% genes.

Experts' Reviews

There are good points to this natural and pure approach to healthy eating. The program's goal is to promote the consumption of food items like whole grain products, fruits, vegetables, complex carbohydrates, healthy fats, and lean protein. However, just like other programs, it isn't perfect. Some experts have criticized certain aspects of this program.

According to Roberta Anding, MS, RD, the spokeswoman of American Dietetic Association, you can follow the basic rules and use its meal suggestions but skip the nutrition advice from the program. Following the program's nutrition and supplement advice could lead to certain deficiencies. Anding added that there are studies that prove that small amounts of alcohol, which is discouraged in this program, could be helpful as it can be cardio-protective. She further stresses that small amounts of saturated fat are unavoidable and not totally harmful to one's health.

Another nutrition expert, Priya Kathpal, says the same thing about the program. According to Kathpal, following a program without an expert's guidance could lead to deficiencies. For her, it's also not feasible to always have organic produce since the availability of organically grown fruits and vegetables vary from one place to another. This program, in her opinion, is costly since organically grown products cost more than those that are not.

Other issues being raised in this program is its restrictive structure, which can also raise issues on its sustainability. Programs like the Eat Clean diet can be difficult to follow in the long run.

Why Follow the Diet?

The expert's review stated that nutritional deficiencies may take place while following this diet. However, studies have shown that the deficiencies only take place when the dieter does not follow a nutritionally balanced meal plan.

As a matter of fact, nutritional deficiencies are more prevalent to people who are following other diet programs. Other dietary programs that don't discourage the consumption of processed foods are more likely to cause nutritional deficiencies. Most processed products go through rigorous treatments before being sold in the market. According to several studies, extensive processing does not just add harmful substance but also removes the nutrients contained in foods. Some diet experts even believe in the efficiency of the program when it comes to weight loss and health improvement.

Do You Want to Be Leaner and Healthier?

If you are aiming at becoming leaner and healthier, then this diet is a good choice. It recommends foods that are rich in antioxidants, vitamins, fiber, and healthy fats. These foods are also preservative-free, which makes them healthier options. Plenty of dieters have already experienced overall improvement of their health condition by following the diet.

Eating small meals frequently can help your reduce cravings and hunger. You won't also gain extra pounds because you will consume less fat and sugar. With these, you can lose 3 pounds a week while practicing the diet. These are excess and unwanted fats that you can get rid of while following this dietary program. Once you achieve the body and weight that suits you, you will be able to maintain it by continuing the diet.

Is It Right for You?

Because you have the freedom to choose your own food, the Eat Clean diet is relatively safe for those who are on a vegan diet or are vegetarians, as well as those with allergies, and/or those with certain dietary restrictions. Diabetics and people with special health considerations should consult their physician for some adjustments.

You can make the easiest transformation from being sluggish to being energetic by simply eating clean. Fitness professionals even find the diet a brilliant way to change a person eating habits on a daily basis.

How to Start Eating Clean

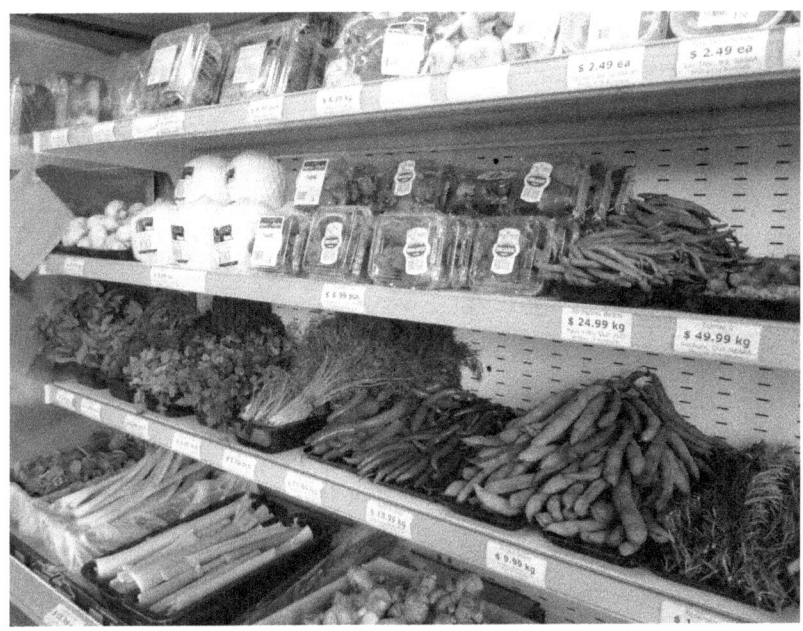

The previous chapters have provided you with sufficient information regarding the Eat Clean diet. Now, you may have probably decided that it is good for you, it's what you need to start a healthier life, and the benefits of the program outweigh its flaws. However, before you jump into the bandwagon of this eating program, it is necessary to learn the steps on how you can get started with it.

Here is a guide on how you can start eating clean:

1. Get Rid of Unclean Foods

Go over your cupboard and pantry and get rid of all of your unclean foods. These include processed and canned goods, refined flours, simple carbohydrates, trans fats, foods with preservatives, and food products with artificial additives and sweeteners. Doing this provides you a fresh start.

2. Shop for Clean Eats

Once you have cleared your freezer, cupboard, and pantry of those unhealthy foods, it's time to replenish your stocks with healthier alternatives. When shopping for clean food, always remember the principle of the Eat Clean diet. To avoid forgetting which clean foods you should buy, preparing a shopping list will help. Save time by shopping for meals good for a week or two. When you do this, don't forget to include a list for your snacks. The local farmer's market is a good place to shop for natural, organic produce.

3. Go to the Periphery of Grocery Stores

The periphery is a section in the grocery store where you will find the healthiest and most natural products. It normally displays whole grain baked goods, fresh produce, meat, dairy products, dried fruits, and other healthy essentials. Make sure that you concentrate on shopping in the periphery to make the most out of the healthiest products offered by the grocery store.

4. Prepare the Meals

If you have already shopped for clean eats, it's time to do the real work – preparing for clean meals. You don't have to fret if this is your first time to do this. There are free resources online that you could turn to for help. The popularity of this program has paved way to a number of meal ideas that you can try.

5. Start with Lemon Water

Nutrition experts recommend the consumption of lemon water first thing in the morning. You can slice a lemon and squeeze half of it into a cup with warm water. This drink will help improve digestion, get rid of toxins, and set the tone for the day. You will be able to make the right start by consuming lemon water in the morning.

6. Cook in Batches

One of the best ways to make sure that you always have healthy meals for yourself and your family is to cook in batches. You can schedule a day or two to do this. You may want to seek your family's help in preparing these meals. Not only will this be a good bonding activity for everyone, it will also help each member to see what's in their food.

7. Don't Forget the Food Combinations

One of the best ways to start eating clean is to combine lean protein with carbohydrate. You can combine fish or meat with grains, wheat, potatoes, or other fruits and vegetables with starchy carbs. The protein will take care of making you feel full for longer periods, and when it's combined with carbs, your insulin levels are less likely to rise.

8. Enjoy Your Meal

The Eat Clean diet is not just an eating program. It is a way of life that also advocates a good approach towards food. So, after you have done the hard work, it's time to sit down and enjoy your clean food.

9. Map Out Your Goals

Set your goals every week or every month and make sure that you continue to practice the changes that you have already made. You should also keep track or take note of the progresses and little successes that you make every week. For instance, you will try to achieve restocking your fridge next week or losing 8 pounds next month.

Starting to eat clean is a lot easier than following other diet programs. There are no strict dieting rules to follow and you can gradually make changes in your eating habits according to your convenience and lifestyle.

Different Ways to Eat Clean

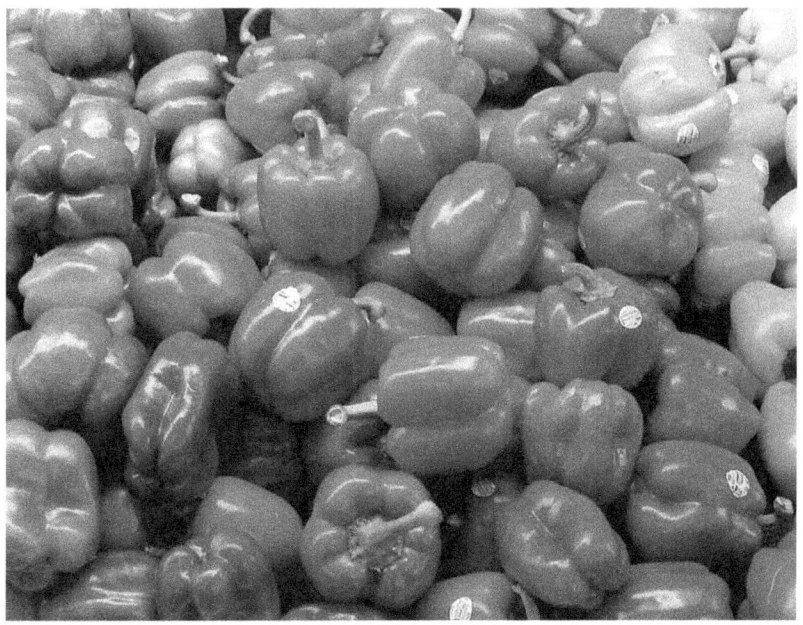

One of the best things about the Eat Clean diet is that it's flexible enough to suit the dietary needs and preference of every person. It can be safe for anyone, whether you're a vegan or a huge meat lover. Unlike other diet programs, the Eat Clean diet allows you to experiment with your food choices, giving you the freedom to choose and to mix and match.

The following are just some of the numerous ways on how you can eat clean. Remember that these are just suggestions. If you have certain health considerations, it would be better to consult a nutrition expert and your doctor.

1. Reduce Your Alcohol Intake

While there are studies showing that alcohol could promote blood thinning, raise your levels of HDL or good cholesterol, and reduce one's risk of dementia and Alzheimer's, the Eat Clean diet doesn't promote the consumption of alcohol. If you can't resist a drink or two, one thing that you can do is to stick to the recommended amount – one glass of wine for women and two glasses for men in a day.

2. Keep Your Sugar Intake under Control

A diet high in sugar is associated with risk factors for high cholesterol level and heart disease. According to the American Heart Association, the recommended amount of added sugar for a person is 6 teaspoons per day for women and 9 for men.

3. Decrease Salt Intake

A high intake of salt is one of the culprits of cardiovascular diseases such as hypertension and stroke. One of the ways to cut down your salt intake is to limit your consumption of processed food products. The majority of processed foods are high in salt. Another trick to curb your salt intake is to cook your meals at home and add flavor to food by adding herbs and spices instead of table salt.

4. Reduce Your Intake of Saturated Fat

Saturated fat could raise your LDL or bad cholesterol. Common sources of saturated fat include whole milk, cheese, butter, and animal fat. You can reduce your intake of saturated fat by opting for healthier alternatives. These include nuts, avocados, and olive oil.

5. Choose Whole Grain

In contrast to refined grains, whole grains contain necessary nutrients plus fiber. They make you feel fuller for a longer period, so frequent eating of unhealthy stuff is controlled.

6. Choose Healthier Alternatives

This means that instead of eating canned peaches, choose the fruit. If you want to have strawberry jam, it is best that you make one using fresh strawberries and other all-natural ingredients. In buying vegetables such as spinach, avoid the frozen ones with sodium-rich sauces. Prepare soup from the clean ingredients that you have in your pantry instead of using dehydrated soup mix or canned soup.

7. Stop Eating Out

You can maintain clean eating if you stop dining at restaurants or fast foods chains. Reducing the number of times you eat out is essential in this diet. If you eat out you will never know if the meals you consume at restaurants are clean. When you prepare your own meals, you are guaranteed that every ingredient is natural and safe.

8. Determine the Right Water Intake

The previous chapters have already stated that drinking a lot of water is essential in this diet. A lot of water often means 8 glasses in a day. However, you can also consume some healthy beverages in addition to the 8-ounce glasses of water every day. You just need to drink only when you are thirsty and sip it instead of gulping. It is also wise that you drink water before meals as this will help you eat less. You also need more water if you are engaged in physical activities every day or if you live in a hot climate. Lastly, prioritize eating foods with high water content such as watermelon, yogurt, and lettuce.

9. Go Organic

The healthiest type of fruits and vegetables are those that are organically grown. Go organic and if possible, grow your own foods at home. You may grow an organic garden containing the fruits, vegetables, and herbs that you typically consume. This will ensure that you won't consume pesticide residues that are often present in store-bought foods. Bear in mind that the pesticide residues are greatly associated with the development of certain life-threatening medical conditions such as cancer. Grow vegetables that are known to have the highest pesticide residues such as sweet bell peppers, spinach, cucumbers, and lettuce.

10. Eat When You're Hungry

The diet recommends eating small meals frequently in a day, and you should eat some of these meals when you're hungry. Never starve yourself and eat as you normally do but only in small portions of healthier foods. You can have some nuts or fruits for snacks every time you feel hungry. Don't allow yourself to feel extremely hungry and impulsively feed yourself with unhealthy foods just to satisfy the hunger.

There are still more ways that you could start eating clean. The choice is totally up to you. So, choose those ways that suit your needs and your new lifestyle at the same time.

Common Clean Eating Mistakes

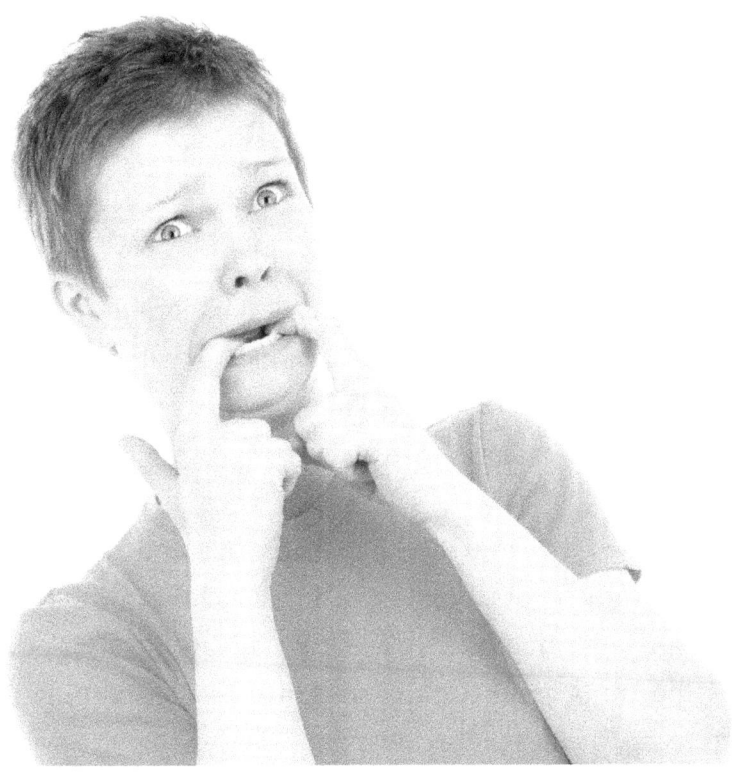

You stick to the program, religiously follow its principles and rules, and then suddenly figure that there is something wrong. You may not feel the way other dieters also using the Eat Clean diet feel. You swear that you did every possible thing to counteract anything that could backfire at your Clean Eating efforts, and still, you feel unhealthy.

If you've been feeling this way since starting the program, then you either did not pay much attention to the guidelines of this eating program or committed one or a few of these common Clean Eating mistakes:

Choosing the Wrong Kind of Fat

Because the Eat Clean diet is not a typical eating program, it promotes eating a well-balanced meal. This means a balanced combination of carbohydrates, lean meats, and fat is recommended. However, you should know that while fats are needed by the body for insulation, brain function, hormone health, and the like, indulging with this food group, especially the wrong kind, could turn your health back to its former, sorry state.

Not all fats are created the same. There are trans, saturated, and unsaturated fats. What you should include in your meal plans are foods that contain unsaturated fats. The two other fats, the trans and saturated fats, are responsible for the increasing incidence of lifestyle diseases, so limit your intake of them. Consume more unsaturated or healthy fats that can be found in nuts, legumes, olive oil, and avocados.

Mindless Fruit Eating

While fruits and vegetables take a huge part in the Eat Clean diet, one shouldn't assume the idea that overindulging on these won't do any harm. The key to succeeding in any eating program is moderation. There are fruits that, when taken beyond the recommended serving, could take a toll on your health, especially if you have certain conditions that require limitations on sugar intake. The right amount of fruits and vegetables that is ideal for you may depend on your weight, weight loss goals, health condition, and other factors.

If you are one of the dieters who eat more fruits than vegetables, then you should start making some changes. Keep the sugar levels low by reducing your fruit intake such as substituting apples with celery stick.

Loading on Starchy Carbs

Just like fats, carbohydrates are also not created the same. It is sub-divided into two groups: the complex and simple carbohydrates. If you plan to start eating clean, then you should ditch your habit of loading up on too much starchy carbs. Compared to complex carbohydrates, starchy or simple carbohydrates don't contain as much as fiber and nutrients as unprocessed ones. Because starchy carbs often lead to a sudden surge and crash of your glucose level, you end up snacking all throughout the day. As mentioned in the previous chapter, it is best that you pair starchy carbs with lean protein to stabilize your insulin levels.

Consuming Protein Bars

Protein is important, no doubt about it. While most protein bars do have protein in them, they are still not considered to be 100% healthy and acceptable for the Eat Clean diet. One reason is the added sugar and other additives in these bars. Most of the protein bars available in the market have plenty of carbs and ingredients that are hard or impossible to pronounce. In order to eat clean, you should stop consuming protein bars.

Skipping Breakfast

Skipping breakfast is another common mistake that you should avoid. Bear in mind that breakfast is the most important meal of the day. When you skip breakfast just because you're in a hurry, you'll end up hungry before lunch and eating sugary muffins or other unhealthy foods. You can have a vegetable smoothie for breakfast as it will only take a few minutes to prepare the drink.

Not Eating Enough Food

Not eating enough food won't make you slimmer and healthier. Although it is true that you won't ingest calories while starving yourself, the effects are only temporary. If you continue to deprive your body with the amount of nutrients it needs, your metabolism will slow down. This will stop your body from burning energy and encourage it to store more fat. In other words, you will become very tired, oversleep, and weak. Make sure that you eat according to how this diet should be practiced.

These are the most common mistakes of people following the Eat Clean diet. Many people think that just because the food is low in calories, it's also healthy, which isn't necessarily true.

Preparing Foods Inappropriately

Never peel your fruits and vegetables especially if they are organically home-grown. The skin of fruits and vegetables are packed with nutrients that are too significant to miss. You should also refrain from boiling your vegetables and instead pan steam them. Another inappropriate way of preparing foods is to slice fruits or vegetables too early. If you let the sliced items sit for a longer period, the nutrients will start to disappear. Make sure that you prepare them not too early before they are taken.

When picking out food items, one of your primary considerations should be the nutrients that you can get out of it. The number of calories is important, especially if you're aiming to lose weight, but then the nutrient content should come first before that

Essential Grocery List for Clean Eating

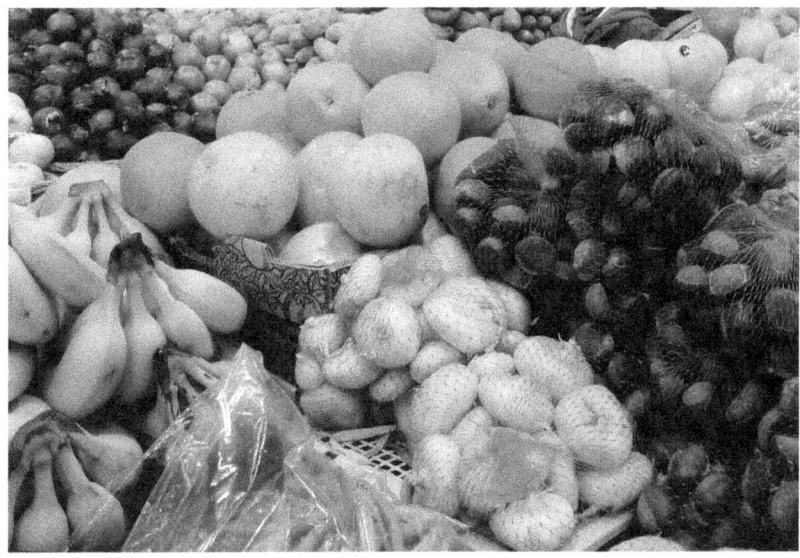

Shopping for the essentials of the Eat Clean diet can be tricky. For some people, just the thought of replacing all their "unclean" food scares them. This overwhelming reaction is normal and is typical among those who are still on the adjustment phase of the program. If you find yourself in this stage, you don't have to fret. Here are some tips to help you get at ease with the process:

Take Your Time

You don't have to rush. Take your time in examining each item in your pantry. Bear in mind that it is not necessary to eliminate all the bad foods. You can just eliminate the worst items first, and then gradually get rid of the others in the next few days or weeks. Once you have already discarded some of the worst food items, you may start making your grocery list.

Prepare Your Grocery List

Preparing your grocery list is the start of this Clean Eating journey. Allow yourself to make necessary adjustments, especially if you personally feel that it is a major transition and you want to tackle it step by step. It's okay to miss an item or two. The important thing here is to stick to the basic principle of the program.

Below are some of the essential items that you should consider when going shopping for this Eat Clean diet:

<u>**Grains and Protein**</u>

- Brown rice

- Millet

- Black beans

- Pinto beans

- Lentils

- Chickpeas

- Raw almonds

- Raw cashews

·Sunflower seeds

·Walnuts

·Almond butter

·Cannellini beans

·Flax seed

Vegetables/Herbs

·Kale

·Lettuces

·Onions

·Garlic

·Cilantro

·Parsley

·Tomatoes

·Broccoli

·Potatoes

·Fennel

Condiments/Flavoring

·Extra virgin olive oil

·Coconut oil

·Sesame oil

·Black pepper

·Pink Himalayan salt

·Hot sauce

·Turmeric

·Cayenne

·Gomasio

·Cinnamon

·Red pepper flakes

·Maple syrup

·Tamari

·Stevia

·Dijon mustard

·Apple cider vinegar

·Red wine vinegar

Fruits

·Lemons

·Avocado

·Apples

·Bananas

·Melon

·Grapes

·Berries

Snacks

·Raw chocolate

·Coconut ice cream

·Tortilla chips

·Popcorn

·Pretzels

·Dairy-free cheese shreds

·Frozen fruits for smoothies

·Bagged frozen veggies

·Organic canned soups

Beverages

·Coconut water

·Herbal teas

·Almond or hemp milk

Pick the Fresh Ones

You will know if the fruit or vegetable is fresh through its appearance and texture. The fresh ones are typically more flavorful and rich in nutrients. Choose fruits and vegetables that are free from bruises and spots. Also make sure that they have smooth skin and don't have cracks. If you make sure that the items are fresh, you will be able to make the most out of their nutrients.

Identify What Foods Are Processed

There are certain food items and cooking ingredients that are processed but are not marketed as such. There are also grocery items that are minimally processed such as those cooked at high temperature for too long. There are also items that are extensively processed such as those with many ingredients. Exercise care in choosing the items that you put in your cart. Always remember that it can be difficult to find items that have not went through processing or treatments.

Avoid Natural but Poor Quality Products

These are grocery items that are raised in soil that are fed with toxic pesticides and fertilizers. It also includes livestock that are fed with hormones to speed up growth and antibiotics to increase immunity from diseases. Make sure that you choose products that have been farmed properly or organically. If you choose poor quality products, it will still defeat the purpose of having this diet.

Make the Diet Work for You

One of the secrets in being able to continue this diet for longer periods is to make it work for you. Choose food items included in the list that suit your taste. This will make your dietary and lifestyle changes not too difficult to follow.

If you are just starting to follow this diet, you need not overwhelm yourself by cooking fancy meals. You can start with simple recipes that only require a few ingredients. This will make things easier especially if you don't normally cook, or you're new in the diet.

Clean Eating Meal Ideas

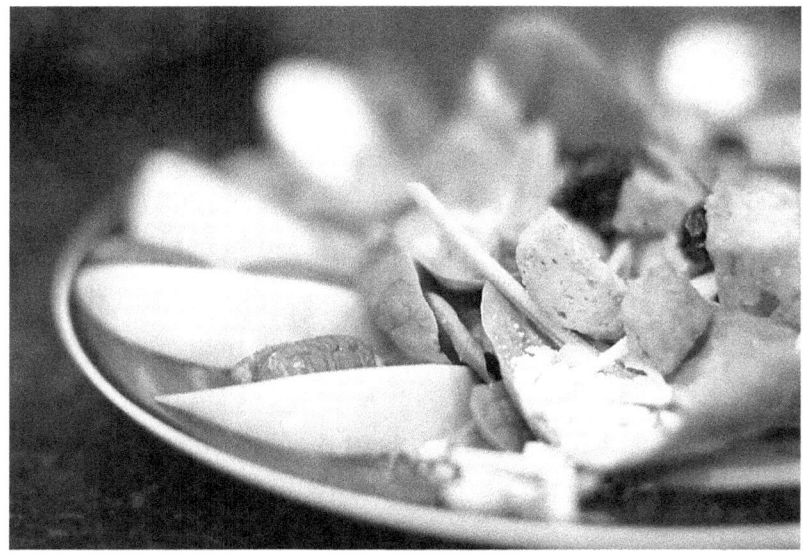

Look good, feel great, and live a healthier life with these easy to prepare Clean Eating meal ideas.

Breakfast Meals

Pumpkin & Apple Waffles

This breakfast meal only takes about 10 minutes to prepare. You just need to use wheat pastry flour, baking powder, cinnamon, and nutmeg in a bowl. Use separate bowl to mix egg and sugar. You may mix the two bowls and add pumpkin puree and chopped apples. Use waffle iron to cook the mixture. Serve with maple syrup and the remaining chopped apples.

Banana Walnut Protein Pancakes

In a shallow bowl, mash bananas until you achieve a smooth consistency. Add the walnuts and set the mixture aside. In another bowl, beat the egg whites until stiff. Get prep bowl and combine dry ingredients such as ground flax, wheat germ, ground cinnamon, protein powder, sea salt, and rolled oats. In a bowl, combine the mashed bananas, walnuts, egg whites, and the wet ingredients. Add the dry ingredients. Mix them well. Over medium heat, heat a skillet and coat it lightly with oil. Pour around ¼ cup of the batter and cook each side well. Do this until all the batter has been cooked. Serve it with the maple syrup or Greek yogurt.

Lunch Meals

Potato & Egg Italiano Sandwich

Beat egg whites and whole eggs in a bowl. You may then sauté the diced potatoes with water and olive oil at medium heat. Add chopped onion, garlic, and red pepper after 5 minutes. When the potatoes are soft, pour the egg mixture, flip, and cook. Combine black pepper, olive oil, cheese, and basil in a separate bowl. You may the spread the basil-cheese mixture on the whole-wheat Italian roll, add the egg mixture, spinach leaves, and tomato slices.

Turkey and Chickpea Burger

It can take about 25 minutes to prepare this delicious burger. The first thing that you need to do is combine cumin, Worcestershire sauce, scallions, pepper, salt, and chickpeas in a food processor. Make sure that the mixture turns smooth before transferring it to a large bowl and adding turkey. Mix it by hand and then divide it to form patties. You may cook the patties over medium heat in a nonstick skillet for 6 minutes. Once the patties are cooked, fill in the whole-wheat bun with it. Top with tomatoes, spinach, onions, and Dijon mustard.

Dinner Meals

Salsa Chicken

Using a crock pot, mix boneless and skinless chicken breast, diced tomatoes, salsa, granulated garlic, red pepper flakes, black pepper, and cayenne pepper. All the ingredients should be combined and cooked for at least 7 hours in a crock pot. Shred the chicken in the pot. Let it cool and transfer in a separate container. You may add sliced onion, bell pepper, cilantro, and lime to enhance the flavor.

Sautéed Vegetables

This delicious and simple recipe can be prepared in around 25 minutes. The cooking process is easy as all you need to do is sauté chopped yellow onion, green onion, red peppers, fresh mushrooms, and garlic. Make sure that all ingredients are diced before you start cooking them.

Snacks

Carrots with Avocado Dip

You can have a tasty and healthy snack by preparing carrots with avocado dip. Make the dip first by combining green peas, chopped avocado, garlic, and lime juice. Once you achieve your desired consistency, add salt, pepper, and hot sauce to taste. You may then use the dip with the sliced carrots to have a healthy snack.

Sweet Potato Crunches

Cut the peeled sweet potato into julienne strips. Place the strips in a bowl and drizzle with olive oil. You may then bake it for about 30 minutes until crispy. You may discard the overly browned potato strings and consume the yellow-brownish strips.

Soups

Thai-Inspired Tomato Soup

Prepare cherry tomatoes, water, extra-virgin coconut oil, chopped lemongrass, lime juice, minced ginger and garlic, and salt. Combine the ingredients in a blender and blend until smooth. You may top with basil before serving.

Broccoli Soup

Boil cauliflower for about 10 minutes and then add broccoli. Cook for another 3 minutes until the vegetables are tender and soft. You may drain and set the vegetables aside once they're cooked. Get another pot and sauté onions at medium heat for 3 minutes. Add garlic and after 2 minutes, add basil, beans, and broth. Remove it from the heat after boiling and then add the softened vegetables. Make a puree out of the mixture by using a blender or food processor. You may then garnish with cheese, toasted pine nuts, salt, pepper, and the remaining broccoli cuts.

Salads

Chickpea Salad

In a medium-sized bowl, mix chickpeas, chopped red peppers, kalamata olives, and cherry tomatoes. You may also add chopped parsley, scallions, and garlic. . Add some salt and pepper to taste, drizzle with olive oil, and add the fresh lemon juice. Mix them well together. Serve.

Arugula with Grape and Sunflower Seed Salad

This salad recipe is rich in antioxidants and vitamin E. To prepare this, just combine red wine vinegar, honey, maple syrup, and stone-ground mustard. You may then gradually add grapeseed oil while stirring. In a separate bowl, combine baby arugula, red grapes, sunflower seeds and chopped fresh thyme. You may then mix the vinegar mixture with the arugula. Add salt and pepper to make the salad a lot tastier.

Side Dishes

Lemon Garlic Asparagus

Preheat oven to 405 degrees F. Line the cookie sheet with aluminum foil. Arrange the asparagus on it. Drizzle the asparagus with olive oil and then squeeze lemon on it. Sprinkle with salt, pepper, garlic, and dehydrated onion. Bake for 8 minutes. Let it cool then serve.

Easy Tahini Detox Carrot Slaw

In a bowl, combine tahini, lemon juice, maple syrup, curry powder, black pepper, salt and garlic powder. Make sure that you whisk the mixture well. In another bowl, combine the carrots, raisins, and pumpkin seeds. Pour the dressing over the carrot mixture. Toss well until it is well coated. You may then pour the mixture to another bowl and let it sit in the fridge for an hour then serve.

Conclusion

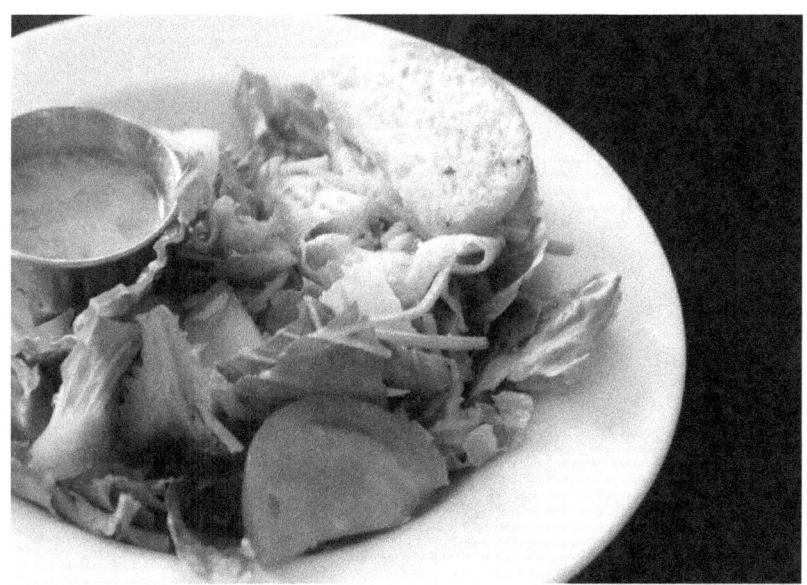

In this fast-moving society, one of the things that is often neglected is our health. Almost everyone is chasing their dream, and they place high importance on every second. It is no longer a surprise why many people opt to settle for processed and fast meals rather than going slow and enjoying homemade, natural and organically grown food and food products. However, you pay the price for it. The increasing incidence of lifestyle diseases including diabetes and heart diseases demonstrates how unhealthy foods can harm the body. True enough, you become what you eat.

The alarming incidence rate of these diseases has encouraged many people to change their eating habits. It has paved way for many health and fitness enthusiasts to come up with diet and eating programs that cater to the health needs of people. One of these programs is the Eat Clean diet.

This program is far from perfect, yet it lays down what a healthy diet should be comprised of. It stresses the importance of consuming whole foods in their most basic or natural form. Although this program isn't created for those who want to lose weight, it provides a good foundation for everyone who wants to start living a healthier life.

Like other programs, it isn't free from criticisms. It has its flaws and its unique set of benefits to the consumer. The choice is totally up to you. You could either focus on its benefits or turn it down due to its flaws. Just like the freedom it gives you in choosing your own food, the choice of whether to take part in this revolutionary program is also in your hands. Besides, it's your health. No one can decide for it other than yourself.

About the Author

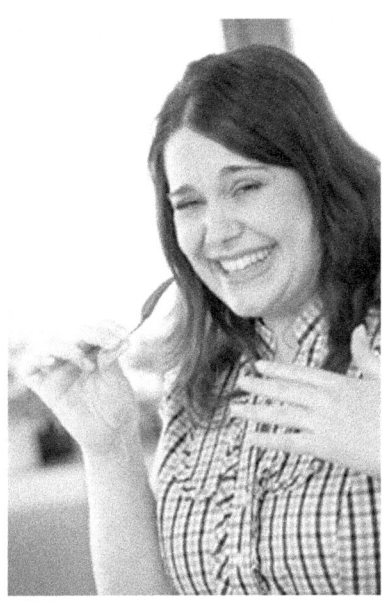

Amelia Simons is a food enthusiast, wife, and mother of five. Frustrated with traditional dieting advice, she stumbled upon the Paleo lifestyle of eating and has never looked back. Without bothering to count calories or stress about endless hours of exercise, eating the Paleo way enabled Amelia and her husband to effortlessly drop pounds and lower their cholesterol.

Amelia now enjoys sharing the Paleo philosophy with friends and readers and finding new ways to turn favorite recipes into healthy alternatives.